T0065283

Can't Scratch That Itch

Can't Scratch That Itch

**A Handbook for People Whose Arms
and Hands Don't Work Anymore**

Tim Griffin

authorHOUSE®

AuthorHouse™
1663 Liberty Drive
Bloomington, IN 47403
www.authorhouse.com
Phone: 1 (800) 839 8640

Published by AuthorHouse 09/03/2015

ISBN: 978-1-5049-4856-2 (sc)
ISBN: 978-1-5049-4857-9 (e)

Library of Congress Control Number: 2015914514

Table of Contents

Dedication – to Karen

Prologue

6 AM – I gather myself on the bed and flop over and notice Karen is already out of bed but decide to lay there for a few more minutes. 6:30 AM and I kick off the covers that I have covering my legs, rotate a bit to the left and lean forward forcing my legs over the side and stand up. Our day begins. Looks a bit like a whale on the beach trying to stand up on its tail.

I walk into the den where my wife is having a coffee and looking at her iPad. "Can you pull this out for me?" "Sure", she says – "I prefer it when you kiss me when you do that – I don't feel so cheap" I say smiling – I walk into the attached bathroom, pee and return to the den. "Would you like your coffee now?" "Sure" – "I will get it for you" – she gets up and goes in the kitchen – I then bend over my laptop which sits on a small ottoman and with my index finger let my finger fall down on the on/off switch. I sit down in front of the laptop with my hands balanced on my knees and allow my middle finger to drop on the keys that are necessary to get my morning paper up on the computer.

Karen comes back in carrying my coffee – adjusts the cup holder on my computer table which is next to me – puts the cup in the holder – adjusts the straw so that I can easily reach it – walks around the ottoman – bends over and gives me a kiss – says "I love you" – sits back down to resume her reading and finish her coffee.

We both spend the next 30 minutes or so looking at our computers and watching the Today Show – "What would you like for breakfast?" "I'd like a smoothie if that would be okay" "no problem" and she gets up again, heads to the kitchen while I continue reading the paper. "It's ready". So I get up from the sofa where I'm sitting and head into my chair at the table where a beautiful fruit smoothie arrives. "Would you like your coffee in here?" "No thanks, I'm great" – and so she begins making her yogurt and fruit dish and comes and sits beside me.

"I need to go use the toilet now – will you listen for my call?" "Sure" as she continues to finish her breakfast. So I head into the master bath – manage to get my pajama bottoms off – use the toilet – clean my butt thanks to the bidet– go in the closet and open the bottom drawer with my toe – reach my foot in and pull up cargo shorts out and onto the floor – kick them back through the bedroom and into the living area and into the kitchen where Karen helps me pull them on and buckles them and zips them up. "Is there anything else you need right now?" "No, I'm good" I then head back into the den – lean over the remote control and drop my finger down to change the channel to the golf channel. My wife now knows that she has some time to herself to finish her coffee, clean up the kitchen and perhaps respond to some emails.

"I'd like my hair washed this morning before we go do anything and a fresh shirt" – so I meet her in the master bathroom – I lean over the sink and she washes my hair, then dries it, then brushes it. "What shirt would you like to wear?" "I think the black T-shirt will be fine" and while I bend over she slides it over my arms and my head and adjusts it. She brushes my hair one more time, puts some toothpaste on the end of my electric toothbrush, wraps my hand around the base, adjusts my hands "is that okay?" "Yes" and pushes the On button. She then starts brushing her teeth and while doing that walks into the bedroom to start making the bed. Comes back into the bathroom, takes my toothbrush and washes it off. "Is there anything else you need right now?" "I don't think so – thank you for everything you've done this morning."

It is only about 7:30 or 8 AM in the morning – by my count there are approximately 22 specific tasks that Karen has performed just for me – I have interrupted what she was already doing at least five times – and she has had to stand up and/or move to another room a combined 7+ times.

It is only 8 AM – want to be a caregiver? I cannot even begin to express my love and appreciation for this woman.

Introduction

"Hope is so important – for me to have hope is not so much that I believe the miracle has to happen to me – however it is critical that I believe that miracles can happen – and I do." Tim Griffin

It is very difficult to explain how different life is when you lose the use of your arms and your hands. Over the past three years, due to the progressive impacts of this Motor Neuron Disease, I consistently have lost the use of my arms and my hands to the point I now have lost the ability to lift, move and/or control those limbs. They hang/dangle from my shoulders with no ability to raise my arms or hands or to use my fingers. (I will talk a little later in the book about how I do use my fingers with the help of gravity and the weight of my arms to manipulate a few things.)

It seems that there is a good bit of literature for people who have lost the use of their legs and technology applied to that lack of function. I have not found a lot of information about how people who lose their hands and arms can go about their daily routines and how they can adapt those routines in the things around them in order to do more things for themselves. In fact, as I've looked for devices, tools and advice it is apparent that more solutions exist for those who lost their arms and hands due to injury than for those of us who have been affected by neuromuscular diseases.

As I begin this writing process my intent is to share some personal experiences and some of the things that we have done to our home to be able to function. Perhaps more importantly, I hope to point out and explain some of the feelings and emotions that go along with functioning when you do not have the use of your limbs and have to rely on other people to help you with your personal needs.

My life today has changed so much. But it is also important to note that the love of my family – my wife who lives with this 24 x 7 and is my constant companion and friend – my daughter who lives nearby and provides help whenever we ask – and my friends who go out of their way to help feed me and help me get around which takes some of the pressure off my wife. These people have made a life that has changed so much so much more tolerable.

I need to say in the very beginning that my life is a good one, a frustrating one, but a very good life. Because of all the prayers, thoughts, and acts of kindness I wake up every day with hope.

An Explanation

I am a male – and there are many references and descriptions that are based on being a male. I hope that some of this will help those who are women but realize that some of what I say here will not be helpful.

For Those Whose Legs Do Not Function

I cannot even imagine what it must be like to lose the ability to use your legs. This handbook does not attempt to prescribe solutions for conditions with which I have no experience.

A Tribute

To all those who have lost their limbs and/or the use of their limbs while serving in the Armed Forces. My thanks go to you and my heart goes out to you and your families. My appreciation for your sacrifice cannot be put into words. An inordinate percentage of ALS patients are former military.

Chapter 1

About the Condition

Motor Neuron Disease is a condition that affects approximately 5000 people in the United States every year. Approximately 30,000 people in the United States are living with the disease. You can do the math – within 3 to 6 years most people who have this disease are gone. If you Google Motor Neuron Disease (MND) you will see the following description:

"A **motor neuron disease** (**MND**) is any of five <u>neurological disorders</u> that selectively affect <u>motor neurons</u>, the cells that control voluntary muscle activity including speaking, walking, swallowing, and general movement of the body. They are <u>neurodegenerative</u> in nature, and cause increasing disability and, eventually, death.[1]" Wikipedia

MND has a number of variations. Most people are aware of ALS (which stands for amyotrophic lateral sclerosis) and is what we commonly refer to as Lou Gehrig's disease here in the United States. There are a number of other variations like primary lateral sclerosis, progressive muscular atrophy, and others. Most other countries refer to all of these diseases under the broad category of MND.

Just a brief history about my disease progression –

In the January/February timeframe of 2012 I was on a business trip for three weeks to Dubai. Having had too much to eat and drink over the holidays I was determined to get back into shape for the year. I was staying at a nice hotel next to the sea that had a terrific gym. So between working out and running on the beach along the sea over the next three weeks I lost 17 pounds and was the fittest I'd been in a long time.

H O W E V E R-

Little did I know that two simple things that I noticed during this three-week period was the beginning symptoms of a life-changing disease. The very first thing I noticed was I was having trouble clipping my fingernails. I simply could not push the two ends of the fingernail clippers together with enough force to close the blades and clip off my fingernails. The second was related to my workouts. I was doing repetitions with weights – flies, which means I lie on my back and put weights in both hands and lift them up above my chest and with bench presses where I would lie on my back on a bench and lift the barbell over my chest and do repetitions. This was all very subtle – I mean this was really subtle! I noticed one morning that I was able to do one or two more repetitions with my left hand and arm doing the fly than with my right. I really didn't think a lot about it but it was clear that I had more strength in my left arm than in my right. I also noted that when doing bench presses I was relying more on my left arm than on my right arm. No big deal, right? Wrong!

When I got home from the Emirates I was determined to continue my discipline and really get things ramped up for summer so that I would be in the best condition of my life at 62 years old. We belong to a fitness center here in Denver and so I headed over 3 to 5 times a week to continue my exercise both– aerobic and strength conditioning. One of the things that I was also determined to do was improve my coordination so I began shooting baskets. I've never been a great shot but I do know what I'm doing and how to shoot the basketball. Here was my next aha moment. When I moved beyond the three-point line not only did I have bad accuracy, which was not uncommon, but I could not get the ball to the rim. Now this was getting weird.

In April it was time for my annual physical so I went in to see my doctor. I took a pair fingernail clippers with me to show him that I could not close levers. I also explained to him the challenges with basketball and that I thought that I lost about 25 yards on my drives on the golf course. Being a 62-year-old male, having some of the challenges 62-year-old males have, and watching all the commercials on television about testosterone I asked that he test for that – and he did – and my testosterone was just fine for a 62-year-old man. So he sent me to a hand doctor. She was terrific and did a thorough exam and determined there was nothing structurally wrong with my hand.

The doctor then sent me to a neurologist – I still remember how much I hated that exam – and what has happened since.

It is now June of 2012 and the neurologist performed a number of tests. By the way, I had set aside an hour for this exam and had conference calls scheduled. The exam took three hours. The first thing he did was have me take my shirt and my pants off and just sat there and observed my body – I had no idea what he was doing. Second thing he had me do was walk across the floor on my heels and on my toes – I had no idea what he was doing. Next he checked for strength in my arms, my hands, my legs and my feet. He would have me try to lift my arms, legs, grip his fingers, etc. while he pushed against me with his hands, creating resistance – I still had no idea what he was doing. And then came the really crummy test – the electromyography or EMG. This is a test where they put sensors on your body in two places and send a small shock and measure how long it takes to get from point A to point B. Having this done once or twice is not so awful but having it done for a full hour is really annoying. (I was really getting annoyed at this point and very rudely actually got on my conference call on my cell phone – the neurologist tolerated my inconsiderate behavior) The next test was to check for what I believe is to determine if you have fasciculations. (These are, for lack of a better word twitches, where your muscle is reaching out to your brain and looking for a signal that is not there. I found out later that the reason he was looking at my body so intently was because you can actually see these twitches in your arms and legs and they were obvious to him.) In this test they put a needle in your arm, leg, etc. and are able to detect the fasciculations. I still did not know what was going on.

So at the end of about three hours the neurologist explained to me that I might have a motor neuron disease and that we needed to determine what was going on by eliminating other possibilities so he ordered a set of blood tests that would either confirm or eliminate other possibilities of diseases that look like MND. He used the word ALS for the first time and I began to be angry. (When I got home and shared my experience with my wife she also shared my anger) A couple of weeks later I came back and he informed me that I did not have any of the markers for the other less ominous diseases and he referred me to the University of Colorado Health Sciences for examination by an expert. Now I knew what was going on.

It is now August 2012 – during the summer I continued to travel internationally for my job as a consultant and while in Beijing I had to go down early for a meeting so that one of my colleagues could button my shirtsleeves and my collar. This was going to really affect my life. Oh, and I was still losing yardage at the golf course.

So in my August meeting at the University of Colorado Health Sciences the neurologist examined me and informed me that I most definitely had a motor neuron disease (MND). The exact type yet to be determined as there are no definitive tests for these diseases.

Now let me take you quickly through the progression or more appropriately the digression. All the motor neuron diseases are progressive in nature, meaning that you continue to lose functions and control over your muscles and they continue to atrophy. The pace of the progression is very different in both the pace and the specific limbs and muscles that are affected. These are all factors that determine the exact diagnosis. (In the UK I would probably be diagnosed with "flail arm")

In October 2012 I was riding my bike and got caught in a rut on the road. Previous to this I would have been able to ride through the rut. On this day I just didn't have the strength in my arms and went face first down to the pavement and cracked my helmet, broke my glasses and bloodied my face, my arms and my legs pretty good. That was the last time I rode my bike. Karen had to come and get me.

During the autumn I continued to lose strength and I had informed my boss that I had this disease and that traveling internationally without someone to help me would be difficult so I was basically reassigned to a project where I would be able to work by telephone. (From the very beginning I experienced tremendous support as well as compassion from my colleagues at work but particularly from my boss and his leadership as well as much of the IBM Corporation.)

We also informed our family that we had the disease that did not have a cure and that the outcome would eventually be fatal. So we began the really emotional challenges that those who are diagnosed have to deal with. It is important to note that at this point you don't know whether you have 18 months to live or 10 years – one of the biggest challenges is figuring out and planning for the future when you do not know how long the future is.

We began to make plans not knowing what my rate of progression would be. In February 2013 we joined one of our favorite couples, Linda and Pat, at Bandon Dunes in Oregon for what I assumed would be my last chance to play there – and it was. I was now down to only being able to hit the ball about 100 yards. I also was now using a fork with a big handle that my wife carried in her purse and she needed to cut up my food for me so that I could stab it and eat – but, for most of the world I looked pretty normal.

It's now 2013 of course and by May we went on a great trip with two of our other favorite people to California and I played my last round of golf with Lana and Ridley along with our great friends Bob and Annie at their golf club. I would go up where my friends would hit their drives and then chip up to the green. I was very proud that day as I sunk a 30 foot putt. That was my last round of golf.

In June it was necessary for me to go on short-term disability which would last for six months. By this time I was having trouble dressing myself – particularly hard was getting a shirt over my head so my wife had to do that for me while I could still pull my pants up I wasn't able to buckle them.

In July we moved into a new home. In May we had sold our 80-year-old home in an old part of Denver realizing that it was not adaptable to the future needs we were going to face.

We had been married in the front room of the house and it was our home. There are lots of phases of grief – but it seems like that with this disease you have to deal with all of the stages of grief multiple times. First you get the news – then you lose more strength – then you suddenly lose your career – and you have to change homes – and you give up the things you love to do – this is hard, for both of us.

We were very fortunate to find a new place under construction and make some adaptations prior to the house being finished. We have plenty of room, a beautiful home, and if necessary the ability to live on one level.

Move forward to November 2013 and things are becoming really challenging. While I can still use my fork I have to sometimes stand up at the table to get enough leverage to push it into a piece of steak. My wife begins adapting what she's cooking so that it is easier to cut up and stab. I can still lift a glass but I have to set them down quickly after taking a drink. It was during this time that some of the public embarrassments that happen begin to take place. We are on a wonderful trip to Australia where we used to live and it is Melbourne Cup Day. It's the equivalent of our Kentucky Derby and everyone in Australia seems to take the afternoon off to party, wager and generally have a great time. I spilled three glasses of wine that day – the first happened as a result of me setting a glass of wine down as I would always have done on the table and my hand giving out and pulling the wine over – if I recall the second happened in a similar manner – and in the third instance I was sitting down in our friend's home and the host handed me a glass of wine. I said don't hand me that wine – please don't hand me that wine –oops – it was too late and before he could take it back out of my hand it had fallen in my lap and on the chair and floor. Conway was of course gracious beyond belief. (Much like a person who does multiple repetitions with weights you eventually come to the point where you can't lift at all and of course that happens very quickly with motor neuron disease patients and you can't lift a glass or push a button.)

It is December 2013. Life is really going to change. I cannot bathe myself anymore so my wife now has to shower me and dry me off and put my clothes on. We'll talk a lot more about this later. I will be unable to work as I cannot travel and I cannot effectively use a computer to do the work I have been used to doing and so in December I go on long-term disability. Christmas comes and we have a wonderful time with our family but unfortunately I can't pick up packages or unwrap them. I have a wonderful son-in-law who went with me to Nordstrom's so that I could purchase my wife's gifts, but I can no longer write or sign a card so after choosing the appropriate card for the holidays I scribble my name the best I can. I've made a commitment to my wife that I will not drive if I cannot put the key in the ignition. On January 2, 2014, even using my knee to try to raise my hand with the keys stuck between my index finger and my middle finger I am unable to get the key in the ignition. The day before was the last day I drove.

2014 is really just more of the same – the gradual progression of the disease. We came to the point in the year where I could no longer stab my food and Karen now has to feed me. This is emotionally devastating for both of us – to me it is also one of the biggest challenges we will face. I'll talk more about this later. I gradually lose the ability to push the keys on the computer and the remote control. (What a sad day for a sports junkie and a channel surfer) but I have developed new techniques that work for me now to accomplish both of these things and I'll talk about them in the section on technology.

At this point let me say and reemphasize I have my legs! I can sit down and stand up – I can walk – I can get out of bed by myself – I can sit down on the toilet and get up – I can go for a walk and I do every day – **every day I am reminded how blessed I am.**

So now it is 2015 and I continue to lose small bits of strength in my arms and hands. There isn't much left to lose with my hands and arms so it's hard to say specifically what are those things I can't do this year that I could do last year. Many of our friends have commented that it seems that the disease has stopped progressing – we wish this were the case. We pray that I keep my legs and we pray for those who don't have the use of their legs.

I am not going to attach a picture showing you what my symptoms look like. I would have to show my stomach and that's just not going to happen. Both of my arms dangle from the shoulders and hang limply by my side with the knuckles facing forward and my palms facing backwards. My fingers are curled and look claw like.

Chapter 2

When I Can't Scratch the Itch

"Lord help me to accept the things that I cannot change, the courage to change the things that I can, and the wisdom to know the difference."

There are so many things that you cannot do for yourself as you lose function in your arms and hands but perhaps one of the most frustrating is that of not being able to scratch an itch. When a piece of lint lands on you or you walk through a little spider web or a fly or a mosquito lands on you – you are completely unable to help yourself to remove the object and/ or to scratch. There are times that I think this is the most diabolical and dehumanizing of all the things that happens to us. I am pretty convinced that I have even more phantom itches now than I did before – those mystery itches that have no cause but just want you to touch a spot to make sure there's nothing there.

Obviously if there is someone around you will immediately ask them to help with this problem. But here begins one of the biggest challenges we have – that is to communicate just exactly what you need and where you need it done and with how much force or effort. For those who haven't been through this you cannot imagine how difficult it is for two people to communicate without pointing and without being able to show in any way where the problem is. This simple example is probably one of the best opportunities for me to explain how frustrating and challenging these kinds of communications are for those of us who need help and also for those of you who are trying to help us.

Imagine for a moment that your hands are tied to your body at your waist. I remember as a young boy watching cowboys on TV and the good guy would throw his lasso around the bad guy and pin his arms to his body. That is the sort of restriction that those of us who have lost all muscle and nerve control in our arms and hands experience. Now imagine that a fly or a bug has landed on the side of your head. So here's a real time example of what we deal with. As I was transcribing this text apparently an eyelash fell down on the side of my nose on the top of my cheek. There's no one else home and so I muted my speech to text software and got up and went into the living room where we have a high-back chair and my wife has placed a piece of fabric on the top edge of the chair for me. So I got up from my computer and walked into the living room and scratched away the irritating eyelash and scratched that part of my face so that I was again comfortable. That might not seem like much to people who can just reach up with their finger and flick away something that lands on their cheek but if you can't do that it is important to have a fallback solution. I am very fortunate to still have the use of my legs so getting up and moving in the other room to remove the eyelash was not a problem for me. It is time to remind myself again that I'm blessed and remember how thankful I am that I have the ability to get up and walk. We've actually thought about going to the pet store and buying a post that cats use to scratch themselves and I'm still not sure that is a bad idea as my wife doesn't completely like the idea of me scratching on the back of the chair in the living room.

Now your nose and your cheeks and your forehead are not the only places where we have itches is that we can't scratch. I'm going to cover in detail when we get to the cleanliness section and the toileting section some other techniques for other parts of the body. However, if you are a man, you are probably aware that the area south of our waist itches more than it should. There are absolutely times that there's nothing I can do about it – but as I will tell you later when I'm being showered we use this fabulous brush that provides great relief and comfort.

Chapter 3

Going Commando – or – Doing the Toilet Thing

We might as well tackle early on one of the biggest challenges I face. This is a highly personal issue for all people but it is very personal for those of us who aren't able to do it by ourselves most of the time. As you will hear me say a number of times I am very fortunate that we have the means to purchase certain devices and that we've been creative to come up with some of our own and finally that I have such a wonderful wife who helps me every day.

Beginning with needing to urinate – (there are a number of words I really prefer to urinate but my speech to text never seems to get them right so will stay with urinate for now).

There are a number of different situations that come into play here. What I am wearing, the time of day, and where we are, and who else may be around.

Let me start at home – the easiest situation is in the evening and in the early morning. I wear loose fitting cotton pajamas with a pretty normal fly that we leave unbuttoned when no one else is around. There are times when I am in bed that I'm able to lay on my back, flop my left hand onto my groin area, and I'm not exactly sure how but am able to hold my hand on the side of my fly while I use my core muscles to sort of lean to the left and hope my penis falls out by itself and then I sit up and on occasions my penis falls freely from the fly and I'm ready to stand up and go in to the bathroom. (We have a toilet in our master bathroom that I will talk about later but we also have a powder room just beyond the door of our bedroom where we leave the lid of the toilet up most of the time. Here is a great reversal – trying to reeducate my wife to leave the toilet seat up after she spent 18 years trying to teach me to make sure it was down. When it is not up I am able to balance on 1 foot and lift the toilet seat up with the other foot but it is nice to already have it up.) So I go into the bathroom and am able to do my business, flush the toilet with my left foot or by leaning into the handle with the back of my left hand and bending over which also flushes it and then return to bed.

I mentioned that I'm sometimes able to get my penis out but that much of the time I am not, so I have another technique that I want to share with you. In our den, which is attached to the powder room on the main level of our house I have installed a latch designed for an outdoor gate. (See the attached picture) We have positioned this in such a way that it is just about the same height from the floor as my penis. I simply face my adaptive device and insert the rod through the fly of my pajamas, position the metal rod below my penis and by dipping down slightly and moving ever so gently from left to right I am able to get my penis out from the fly of my pajama bottoms. I get my penis back in my pants by bending over at my waist and pushing my rear end out. That usually works.

I owe the development of this idea of the zipper pull to my friend Bart who helped me by manufacturing the prototype. He welded a base onto a nail that allowed us to screw the device onto a 2 x 4 in my basement. This worked effectively except that it was a bit rough and didn't have the nice machining and smooth edges of the gate latch but it was a very important step in getting the right device.

There is one problem that we've yet to completely solve for and it's a problem for men everywhere even those who have hands. Remember the old rhyme "no matter how much I shake and dance the last few drops go down my pants?" That old adage seems truer than ever for people like me.

Here is where going commando comes into play – I'm going to describe the clothes I wear to make all these activities more efficient. However it is the clothes that I don't wear that really makes this work. So a couple of years ago I joined Jimmy Buffett and I now go commando.

I have taken this technique one step further to use during the daytime. One of the really important things for families that find themselves in situations where one of the family is handicapped is to be able to find

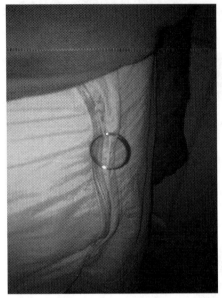

freedom both for that person and perhaps more importantly for the other person in the family, the caregiver. In our situation the biggest problem is that if my wife leaves and I have to go to the bathroom I need to be able to take care of that myself and so we've come up with the following technique.

First of all we found that hiking/ cargo shorts and pants are the easiest for us to adapt/modify. It's really very simple – we purchased a number of key rings that are about three quarters of an inch across – my wife then put one of these rings/ loops through the zipper pull on my pants. We have put these loops on almost all of my pants and shorts (Here are pictures of the loops, and the technique I use to unzip my pants.) In addition to the loop it is also important that you cut out the extra inch or so of fabric behind the zipper so that it does not get in the way when you're trying to get your penis out.

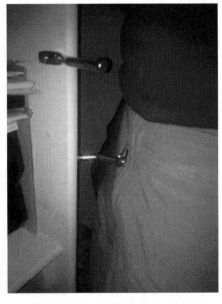

One more really important item which is very personal also. Make sure that you keep your pubic hair closely trimmed. They can definitely get in the way when you're using the technique I described for getting your penis out.

To get your penis back in is usually not that hard. What I found that works is I bend over at my waist and push my bottom out away from me and just bend over and in most cases my penis tucks back in to my pants. Now that's actually the easy part – getting zipped backup is not as easy as getting zipped down. I reverse the zipping down process when getting zipped back up. The problem is that I am unable to zip my pants up all the way because I cannot hold down on the bottom of the zipper as a person who has the use of their hands would normally do. I am only able to get the zipper about halfway. The good news is I can probably answer the door and not get arrested.

So what do we do when we are out in public? It is still very helpful to have the loops on the zippers – but this is where the caregiver comes in. In my case my wife simply has to unzip me and remove my penis from my pants so that I can urinate. She then takes a piece of tissue and wipes off the extra drips, tuck me back in and zips me up. This works best if there's a family bath – Karen still hasn't gotten comfortable going in the men's room.

We also use this same technique when we are home and generally don't have company. It is much quicker than the zipper pull method. (However as I mentioned earlier in the book – when we do this I do smile and ask that my wife give me a quick kiss – that way I don't feel quite so cheap when she unleashes the beast.)

There is a bit more to the story here – so let me share a few experiences with you.

The most advantageous situation is to find a family bathroom. That way my wife can go in with me and we can do the things that are required for me to go to the bathroom and she can wash her hands and we can just simply move on. The one disadvantage that we found in this situation is that people often look at us funny both going in and coming out of the family bathroom. (I guess they think we're joining the mile high club or something) Most of the time we just nod and I smile and in the rare situation now when someone feels the need to make some clever or rude comment one of us is usually able to respond in kind.

When you can't find a family bath it becomes a bit trickier. The way we normally do this is to go up to the door of the men's bathroom and I use my foot and open the door slightly to see if there are other people inside. If I think the coast is clear or if I think I can get in without exposing myself – I have my wife unzip my pants and remove my penis and I simply go in and do my business at the urinal. I do try to be careful to make sure there are not too many people around and of course I am particularly careful to make sure there are no children or women around as I don't want to get arrested.

C A U T I O N: whether you are out and about or at home it is important not to wait until the last minute. As you can tell by all these descriptions this takes more time than if you were doing it yourself. So do yourself a favor and give yourself time.

Going Number Two:

That description of going number one is pretty simple – going number two creates a few more challenges. However, what we've done to accomplish this may be the single most important thing for me. Since this bodily function is so personal and one that I believe most caregivers would prefer not to participate. We have developed the following process.

Again let me say I realize that not everyone may have the means to do this – but we have installed an automatic bidet toilet seat. Ours has a remote control that we place on the floor so that I can operate it with my toes.

Before I get to the step by step process I need to describe for you how I get my pants off. The only pants I can get off by myself at this point are my pajamas. (By the way I am not able to put them back on so it requires having someone home.) To get my pajama bottoms off I simply take my left foot and put it against my pajama bottoms at the ankle level of my right foot and put my weight on the bottom of the leg and push up on my right toe. I do this a couple of times on the right leg and then I do the same thing a couple of times on the left leg and eventually I'm able to pull the pants off. I am fortunate that I have good balance so please be careful with maneuvers like this and some of the others I describe.

Before I sit down on the toilet I get the toilet paper ready. I am able to use the side of my hand – lean against the toilet roll and then I dip my shoulder and roll off the length of paper approximately the distance between the toilet paper holder and the floor. I then put my knees around the paper and squeeze, let my hand drop on top of the role of paper so that it doesn't move, and pull with my knees until the paper is torn away from the role. I then take my toes and fold this length of paper in half to come up with a double layer approximately 16 to 18 inches long.

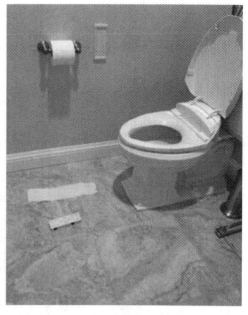

After sitting down on the toilet and doing my business it is time to clean up. Since I don't have any strength in my fingers to even push a button on the remote control I use my toes. (In fact toes and tongue are really important to me for lots of things)

My bidet has some very nice features. The seat and the water are heated and I can actually regulate how warm I want the water. The first step is simple and I press down on the washing button and that sends a strong steady stream of water over my backside and does a very efficient job of cleaning my bottom. Next I push the button for the fan – the fan does not completely dry my backside but it does do a good job of beginning the process.

Now it's time to complete the process. I stand up over the toilet with my legs on either side of the toilet bowl and bounce up and down a bit to try to let any additional water drop off. I then stand up and with my toes I pick up the end of the toilet paper and set it on the right edge of the toilet seat. I try to have about 1 inch of the paper hanging off the edge. I then sit back down with the emphasis on that side of the toilet and with the middle of my bottom strategically positioned so that it will be on the paper and I slide back and forth a couple of times and forward and back a couple of times to remove any additional moisture. For me it is not uncommon for the paper to stick to my bottom so I have to do a few gymnastics of jumping up and down and sometimes sliding forward to catch the paper on the front of the toilet seat – much like a puppy might do to get a dangling piece of poop off the hair on their butt – so that it will drop into the bowl. I then balance on my left foot and flush the toilet with my right foot. (Please don't try this if you don't have good balance – I am leaning against the wall in this picture for balance.) With our new toilets I am able also to lean my left hand against the flush handle and dip my shoulders and flush in that manner. I'm sure that's a lot safer than the one foot method. (I am pretty sure you won't get any of these techniques from your occupational therapist)

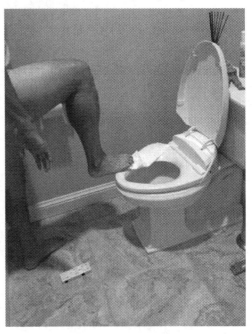

Remember the previous comment about "no matter how much I shake and dance"? Well it definitely applies here and there are always a few drops on the floor. I use my "get pieces of toilet paper off the roll technique" and drop a couple of squares on the floor – wipe up the spots – and put the toilet paper in the toilet. F L US H

I've always done this in private so not even my wife had seen this complete process in person until she took the picture. But for you – here are the pictures of my toilet seat and remote control, the tearing of the toilet paper, the positioning of the toilet paper on the toilet seat.

Of course the challenge is that we are not always home and sometimes we are on the road – here is how we have accommodated being in a hotel room or staying in a friend's home.

We purchased a very simple device on Amazon.com. This device is really a rubber ball that has about a six-inch tube coming from it that turns up at the end at a right angle. Search for "portable bidet."

The problem with this process is that it takes your caregivers full effort and puts them in a position I'm sure they don't enjoy and I don't like either. The first thing you have to do is of course fill the ball with water and I recommend warm water. My wife then has to put the long part between your legs in the front and aim the end of the tube at your rear end. A couple of quick squeezes on the ball should clean your bottom and the excess water drops straight down into the toilet bowl.

After being washed off unfortunately I have to be dried and that is up to the caregiver to do that. I have to say that of all the things that we have to deal with this is the hardest for me. Dignity takes a beating on this one and I am thankful for a loving and caring person because she does everything she can to help me maintain that dignity.

One final note – these bidet toilet seats can be pretty expensive – for the electronic version the cheapest I've seen are around $400 and up to $2000. When we were traveling in Australia last year we stayed for two weeks at friends. Judy and Tom purchased a toilet seat for me that used water pressure without the electronics to clean my rear end. My wife just had to turn the knob and that did the cleaning. Two of the most generous people in the world are our friends Tom and Judy in Australia – Tom may be the most nurturing and caring man I've ever known. We told all our friends in Australia about the toilet seat and the last night there we were having a going away party. Several of the folks thought it would be a good idea to go in and see how this works – so they stood back, turned the knob, and watched as a powerful stream of water shot across the room and nailed the mirror on the other side of the room. It was good fun.

Oh – one other thing. These streams of water can be pretty powerful – so the old saying came to my mind "Friend or Enema"!!

I have one not so happy story. Last summer my good friend Roger and I went up to Moe's barbecue for lunch. Our wives were shopping so we walked. I decided I didn't need to go to the bathroom before we got home because I really didn't want nor was I prepared for my friend to clean my bottom so I decided I would try to make it home to the bidet. I soon found that I could not hold it any longer and unfortunately it wasn't just the need to pee. I pooped my pants. The rest of the walk home sucked beyond belief. We got home – went into the backyard, dropped my pants and Roger hosed me down. There are friends and then there are friends.

Chapter 4

Making the Most of Hygiene

There are so many things that are so personal about all the things that we do in our everyday lives. Going to the toilet was very personal and has not only physical but emotional challenges when you have to be helped. We're going to talk more about eating later and I've already described it as one of the most emotional times of the day for us. But the tasks that we perform to stay clean are the ones where we spend the most time every day. I am going to cover brushing your teeth, washing and combing your hair, shaving, blowing your nose, clipping your fingernails and your toenails, (remember that was the first place I lost function) putting on deodorant as well as the big one – getting showered.

Brushing Your Teeth – I will attach a couple of pictures of the equipment I use and how I use them. Certainly over the last three years my ability to do my dental hygiene has changed. The three key tools to accomplish having clean teeth is a Sonicare electric toothbrush, a toothpick type device that has a bristle brush on it and then some sort of a flossing stick. Here are examples of mine. (See picture of toothpick, flossing stick and toothbrush below)

I can describe the flossing and the tooth pick work very succinctly. At this point I cannot do it by myself so Karen has to do it for me.

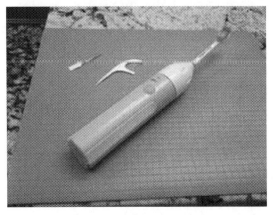

Brushing my teeth is a two-person job even though I am able to still do most of the work myself. My wife puts the electric toothbrush in the saddle of my left hand between my thumb and index finger – she then puts this in the saddle of my right hand making sure all three fingers on the left-hand are on top of the fingers of the right hand.

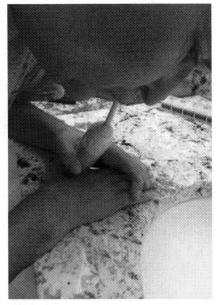

1. I bend over with my arm on the counter and put the toothbrush in my mouth. (She has, of course, already put the toothpaste on.)

2. She then turns on the toothbrush for me and I am able to move my head up and down and backward and forward along the front of my teeth.

3. I then have to hold the toothbrush at the end with my teeth and turn it so that it has the proper angle to do the back of my teeth.

4. I then turn the toothbrush again with my teeth so that I can do the left side of the front of my mouth as I move my head up and down and sideways.

My Sonicare toothbrush has what I believe are four timed periods that last about 30 seconds each. This seems to be adequate time to do all the things I just described above and then it turns itself off. I am usually then able to just let it sort of drop on the counter until my wife is able to wash it off and put it back in the charger. Our terrific friend and dentist Katie says that I do a better job than most people with two hands.

Washing and Combing –

When I shower we obviously wash my hair – but there are many times when we are already up and about and I don't want to go someplace without having my hair washed. I do try to keep my hair trimmed and not too long so I have a haircut at least every three weeks.

On those days when I need to have my hair washed my wife simply rolls a towel and puts it on the edge of the counter in front of the sink and I get my head in and get wet and she washes my hair and then rinses it in the sink. It's very quick and I think takes less than three minutes to do the whole thing. She then dries it and brushes it – since we live in Colorado where it is generally dry my hair is finished drying in just a couple of minutes. This may not have sounded like something we even needed to cover, but if you are at all like me, you still want to look as good as you can and having clean neat hair is important to me. (I also believe it cuts down on itching)

Shaving –

Now this has become an interesting process for us. I can honestly tell you that this was one of the tasks that I was most worried about trusting someone else to do. No offense, but especially a woman.

The easiest and quickest way is to use our electric razor. However, I've never been particularly happy with the shave I get from an electric razor and we have found over the last couple years that when my wife shaved my face with the electric razor it's never quite as close and clean as when we do it with a blade razor.

So we use a Quattro for my shaves. Here is where the fun starts and where you truly need to trust someone and give them time to learn the skills necessary. Just think about it, as a man shaving ourselves we can feel everything that is going on – we can see ourselves in the mirror – we can tighten our face muscles as we need to in order to create the right amount of tension to get a proper shave.

When someone else is trying to shave us they do not have any of that advantage and in the case of my wife she had no experience with this process. So I believe we have both been very patient with each other and she has become amazingly talented at providing a comfortable clean shave. Here's the process:

1. My wife puts a small amount of shaving cream on her hand. (This took some time to learn how much was appropriate) she then applies it around my face and neck and I sort of think she enjoys the art of this.

2. I move my feet so that I position my head in a way that makes it easiest for her to shave me. She begins by shaving below my right side burn, does my right cheek and neck. She then does the left side beginning with my left side burn, then the cheek and neck.

3. Next are the touchy bits – above and below my lip and my chin. She has gotten really good at doing these things and getting them clean-shaven and I think we've done a great job of communicating with each other when I need to tighten the muscle or put my tongue against the inside of my mouth in order to be able to facilitate her shaving me.

The best part of this is when she is done she makes sure that my face is smooth by kissing me. Sometimes it's necessary for her to use the razor a couple more times on my lips and test for smoothness a few more times.

Blowing My Nose –

This is not nearly as fun nor as gratifying as being shaved. In fact, I think this is the hardest task that I am discussing in this section. It is pretty obvious that this is not a pleasant task for anyone. A person that has to face someone – apply just the right amount of pressure on the nostril that you want to close – while making sure that you have the right amount of airflow for the other nostril is really a trick. This is one of those tasks that we perform several times a day and we really do have to be patient with each other.

There is not much to say here other than it is very important to communicate. Let your caregiver know that they have enough pressure on the closed nostril and if you think that things are clear enough on the other nostril so that it can be cleared. We usually use several tissues.

Cleaning My Ears –

Much like your nose this is a bit of a challenge – we use cue tips and tissues. I don't know if it has anything to do with my condition but I create an amazing amount of earwax. Not only is it an issue of hygiene it is also an issue of comfort. When I have wax buildup in my ears you have a natural tendency to want to scratch and/or to clean those ears and I obviously can't do that so this is a really important bit that my wife has to perform for me.

This does not take a great deal of discussion but it does take a lot of communication between us. Having someone poke a stick in your ear makes you very tense. So we do have to communicate about the amount of pressure that she applies.

Here's a hint – every couple of haircuts I have my barber wax my nose and my ears removing all the excess hair. Makes life much easier having all that extra hair gone and it just takes a moment of pain and about $10.

Clipping My Fingernails and Toenails –

Having short fingernails on your hands that are paralyzed is way more important than I would have thought. If my fingernails are too long, due to the fact that my hands and fingers are somewhat claw like, it is not uncommon for me to actually puncture or cut another finger with the sharp edge of the fingernail. Another really important issue is that when using my cellular phone I have to stand above it and let my finger drop down on the buttons using gravity. Because of the technology your actual finger has to touch the button and if the fingernail is in the way it will not activate the button.

Pictures are worth 1000 words for this task and so I will show you one that we have found useful. This is another task, similar to shaving, where you are using something sharp and you are asking a person to perform this from an awkward and unfamiliar position.

Make sure you have really good, really sharp fingernail and toenail clippers. Courtesy of our good friend Lana we have clippers that have an elongated lever on the bottom that improves leverage.

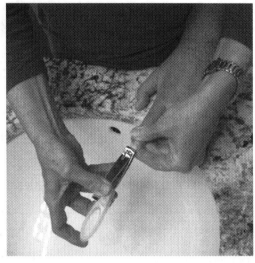

To do my fingernails requires me to stand behind my wife facing her back and she first takes my left hand in her hand and puts it over the sink. She straightens each finger as she clips it. Basically she has my arm between her arm and her side. She then takes my right hand and performs the same function. This all sounds somewhat simple but it is not. It takes real patience for a caregiver to clip someone's nails. I am more nervous during this task than any other.

Toenails are actually easier than fingernails. I sit on a bench facing my wife and she either sits on the floor or on another bench with my foot in front of her. The biggest challenge with toenails is that they tend to be very thick

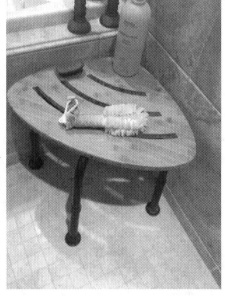

and difficult cut. It is important to have really good, sharp toenail clippers. All of these tasks are finished up with an emery board to help avoid hang nails getting caught on fabric or other items.

Showering –

This is absolutely the best part of my day. I have mentioned this before but we are very fortunate to have had our bathroom built in a way that is accessible for a person with disabilities. At this point we don't have to use those functions

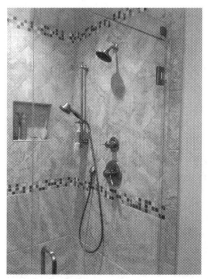

that were designed for a wheelchair but all the doors and all the access places are wide enough and flat enough to accommodate a wheelchair if necessary. Attached is a picture of what our shower area looks like. In a nutshell – we have a wide, 36 inch door – the entrance to the shower is flat having installed what is called a lateral drain – we have a bench in the shower that is portable that we bought at the local store that provides various tools and accessories for the handicapped – and we have both a traditional showerhead that is in a fixed position on the wall as well as a handheld showerhead attached to a flexible tubing. (We have a second home where we did not have the benefit of designing and building the bathroom – we found a showerhead that allows us to retrofit the existing shower with a flexible, handheld showerhead extension similar in function to the one we had installed in our new home at a very reasonable cost.)

I'll share with you a couple of pictures of this process but you will lose some of the impact of the process as my wife said we had to wear our clothes for the pictures. You may now understand why this is the favorite part of my day.

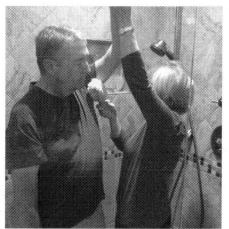

An important part of this task is to have a short handled brush. It not only makes it easier for the caregiver but it also really helps you get clean. Here is the process:

1. The first thing we do is wash my hair – during this process we are using the fixed showerhead.

2. Next my wife soaks up the brush and washes my face – then around my neck and down my chest to my waist –

3. I turn around and face the shower and rinse this off while she is scrubbing my back –

4. I then turn back around and face my wife and rinse off the soapy water from my back while bending over with my arms dangling down. She is able to soap my underarms while I am bending over – I then stand up and she raises one arm at a time and uses the brush to scrub under my arms –

5. Next is for me to raise one leg onto the bench – she soaps my private area and with my foot still up on the bench she uses the brush to scrub on the top of my leg and under my scrotum – I then change to my other leg and she does the same thing –

6. I then turn around and she scrubs my bum and the back of my legs.

7. About once a week my wife washes between my fingers. This isn't as easy as it might sound but it is very important. Since I don't wash my hands on a regular basis the skin gets dry and flaky. My wife will use the brush and spread the fingers and scrub the area between my fingers down to the web part. This exfoliates the skin and makes that area much more comfortable for me.

8. It is time to rinse the soapy water. There is a simple knob to turn that diverts the water from the fixed showerhead to the flexible handheld showerhead. My wife holds up one arm and rinses and then the other arm – I again put my foot up on the bench and she thoroughly rinses that area of my body.

9. Since our shower is pretty big we do the drying inside the shower. We follow the same sequence as when we washed – she raises each arm and dries me off and then I put my leg up on the bench and she dries that area very thoroughly.

Obviously it's now time to get dressed – make sure you have clothes that are very easy to get on and off and are loose fitting. As I mentioned earlier I wear a lot of cargo shorts and pants. I wear pull on cotton T-shirts and golf shirts.

Couple of quick comments about getting dressed – Be Careful! – Make sure you're in a place where you have something to lean against when you're putting your pants on and make sure that your caregiver bends over and doesn't throw their back out helping you to get your pants on. When your arms don't work and you're putting on a T-shirt you have to bend over and let your arms dangle and then have your caregiver put one arm at a time and then pull it over your head and pull it down comfortably. My wife will lift each arm individually and pull down on the underside of the sleeve as well as the cape of the shirt so that they don't bunch up under my armpits. When Karen is putting my pants on I find it helpful to stare straight ahead – this helps me maintain my balance.

I think I mentioned this earlier but it's really important to simplify things. I don't wear underwear – layering shirts is difficult because they bunch up under your arms so try not to do that – and I very seldom wear socks as that makes the caregiver bend over one more time than is necessary.

On a couple of our group trips I've taken advantage of our friends to help me put on a belt or a jacket so that Karen can continue getting ready. I have found that women are much better at this than men and given the choice of Pat or Linda I will take Linda every time.

One of the real challenges in life is to give your caregiver a break so over the last couple of years we have found people to come in and do all these things for me that my wife does on a daily basis. I have hired professional companies who do this as well as actually contracting an acquaintance who did it for me as well. I've had both good and bad results with the professional companies. But the key here is that the process that we use works even when someone else is helping you:

1. The brush is very important as I'm sure the caregiver isn't too excited about touching my private parts.

2. The caregiver gets to stay dressed and can actually stand at the entrance to the shower area and using the handheld showerhead and is able to soap all the parts and then rinse me just as my wife does with the handheld showerhead.

3. The caregiver then towels me off and helps me dress.

(I'm not a particularly modest so I have to say none of this bothers me a lot. It is just the way it is.)

Finally, all of the tasks that I've described regarding showering are very physical for your caregiver. My wife always waits to shower until I'm finished because she has worked so hard to get me showered and dressed that she needs to shower just to cool off. Picking up the arm of a 190 pound man that has no life in it is not an easy task. This takes a physical toll every day on my wife. Please be conscious of the impact that all of these tasks have physically, mentally and emotionally on the people that help take care of us.

One funny story – we moved into our new house two years ago. Over 18 years of marriage we've always enjoyed a Jacuzzi bath with candlelight and some champagne. So here we are two years ago and I haven't tried out the new tub yet so on Sunday night we decided to have our bath. Everything is going great – the Jacuzzi works wonderfully – the champagne is great – candlelight is romantic – my wife is beautiful, and now it's time to get out. At the time I didn't realize it but my arms had weakened to the point that I could not get out of the tub. There I sat in much the same condition that God had made me in the first place. It was late on a Sunday night and we were in a new neighborhood and after Karen tried a number of times to help me get up we realized we were in a real pickle. So I sat there and thought and I thought and finally had Karen put a couple of towels behind me and with one mighty effort I flopped over on my stomach much like a whale would do – smashing my face against the side of the tub and from that position was able to get on my knees and get out of the tub. You can write whatever moral to this story that you want but I can tell you I have not gotten in a tub since.

Chapter 5

Eat, Drink, and be Married

Not sure if my wife would agree with me but I do believe that eating is the most frustrating part of my day. Asking someone to shave you, to blow your nose, pull your pants up are all very personal things. But I have found that because we go about eating very differently and the process of sitting across from someone or next to someone is so different than feeding yourself that you need to think through this process to avoid as much stress as possible.

I will start with drinking because we really have mastered this part of the process. There are a number of things that we do and utilize to make this as easy and allows me to be as self-sufficient as possible. Attached are pictures of the straws that we use and we use a variety of them. We have been able to buy long straws they can actually be clipped off to meet the various needs 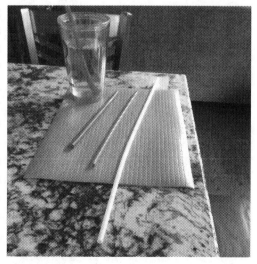 based on length at a local store that caters to people who have handicaps. These are terrific and we keep a supply of them on hand. We've also found a really nice long straw at Starbucks. The straws are longer and a little bit larger in volume than many straws. They also work very well and we often use those at the table. For thicker drinks, for example when I indulge in a milkshake or I drink my soup, there are even thicker straws. So you will see attached the pictures of the straws.

Where I drink is also important – my wife always keeps a full glass of water with a straw on the kitchen counter and one on the bathroom counter. I'm able to go in anytime of the day or night and get a drink of water.

Morning is important to me to have my coffee and read my paper. (I read the paper on my laptop and I'll say more about that later) we have this terrific computer table that I used before I quit working where we keep the telephone. This table rotates and has a holder for a drink cup. My wife brings me my coffee in the morning and puts it in the cup holder with one of the long straws that I 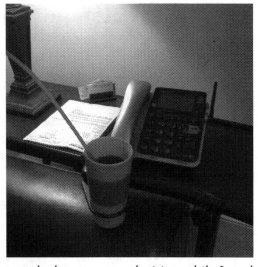 mentioned earlier. I'm able to watch the news on television while I read my paper and enjoy my coffee without troubling anyone else. This is one of the best parts of the day.

When we have company and we are sitting in the living room we have a table next to the chair where I sit and we put my glass of wine or scotch with one of the long straws on the table. This works out very well for me. There was a time six months or so ago that we used a glass that looked a lot like a ball jar with a handle on the side and a lid. We owe the discovery of these glasses to our friend Lyn in St. George. The straw went through a hole in the middle of the lid and I was able to sit in a chair with my arm on the armrest and hold the handle on the mug. I really like this position as I was able to sit in the chair a bit more like a fully able person.

One of the things that we do is use what I would refer to as tumblers. These are glasses that are taller and shaped more like the kind of a glass that you would get a beer in. We have several varieties as well as some insulated cups that do a good job of keeping cold drinks cold and warm drinks warm.

Many of our friends and neighbors have really gone out of their way to accommodate me. Almost all of them now keep straws at their homes and many have actually bought different kinds of glasses with lids so that I can imbibe right along with everyone else. Amazing friends.

Eating isn't quite as easy to do as drinking. One of the things that I try to do is have a healthy smoothie for breakfast and encourage my wife to make soup as much as possible. It really is nice to be able to sit and have my meal and not have to rely on someone else to feed me. (I will talk a bit more about this and the role that our friends have played in giving my wife a break.)

My wife is a really great cook and has always been a very healthy cook. We have lean meat, fish, and my favorite – chicken. She also prepares lots of salads and soups.

Our everyday routine is pretty much a three meal a day routine. Starting with breakfast I have already mentioned that I like to have a smoothie. Mine are made with various berries and bananas and some almond milk. They are delicious and are obviously very good for me. About half the time my wife makes me an omelet. It is usually without cheese but with some type of minced turkey sausage or mushrooms.

Now it's time to talk about how she feeds me. Breakfast is not as big a challenge as some of the other meals because my wife can feed me first and then eat her yogurt.

This may sound really simple but it is not. She will cut my omelet with the fork into pieces that are about 1 inch square. It is important to have the bite large enough that it speeds up the process and gives you something to chew on. My wife sits on my right around the corner of the table from me and using her right hand can feed me. Now here's the tough part. We all like our food seasoned differently – I like a good bit of salt and pepper on my food – as a person who has lost lots of independence we have to sometimes discuss that I want the salt even though she is trying to help me eat a more healthy diet. The other thing that causes some tension for both of us is getting the food into my mouth. Omelets are pretty easy because they can be stabbed. But it really does take some concentration on the part of the caregiver to get the food into your mouth. If they look away and/or are distracted you may find yourself trying to reach or knock the food off of the fork.

Let me take a minute to talk a little bit more about this time and process of feeding someone else. Many times we are alone but a good bit of the time there other people around and there is never a time I am more conscious of my disability than during this time. It is never more visible to others than during this time that I have to rely on another person to do those basic things that each of us do in life. I know going into having a meal I am a bit more conscious than I am at other times. At breakfast, when my wife is not eating at the same time it is generally a pretty good situation. But the one thing that can cause this time to be more stressful is if she looks away at the TV or to talk to someone and seems to forget that I am waiting to have a bite of food put in my mouth. I can only speak for myself but for whatever reason these times are difficult for me. It is also very important to point out that my wife has just prepared my meal and has probably prepared hers and if we have guests their food as well. She then has to take time out to feed me. Not fair.

Lunch is usually a soup or a sandwich. These are pretty simple foods to eat and be fed by another person. We really do try to keep this simple. Remember soups can be consumed with a straw. I can do it myself.

But then there is dinner. It really doesn't matter whether we are eating at home or somewhere else but for the sake of this discussion let's also assume there other people there. The very first thing for me to remember is that my wife, if we are eating at home, has prepared the meal and served everyone. She then prepares my plate – cuts my meat and then prepares her plate. (This is another point where as individuals we do things very differently. I'm a very fast eater and my wife has usually been the last person to finish her plate. Think about what an amazing amount of pressure this puts on my Karen – having to feed me and at the same time trying to feed herself and somehow keep up with everyone at the table.) We have now been functioning like this for well over a year and we continue to get better and better about communicating and about expectations. I can only say how grateful I am that I have a person in my life who is learning to be patient with me and who takes the time and makes the effort to do things differently than she would do them herself.

Just one anecdote here – my wife is a dipper. Let me explain – let's assume for the sake of simplicity that my plate has three items on it. First is some nice brisket that is very tender and has been cooked in a simple sauce with some Worcestershire sauce and other ingredients only my wife would know. We would also probably put a little bit of barbecue sauce on the dinner plate. Next are some cucumbers that are marinated in olive oil along with some spices and finally she's made some marinated mushrooms to go along with the brisket. Now here's the deal – if I were in control of my fork I would cut a piece of brisket, dip once in the barbecue sauce and put it in my mouth. Not my wife – follow this – she might cut off a piece of the brisket with a fork – pull a couple of the mushrooms away from the pile of mushrooms – move the cucumbers around a bit so that some of the oil is separated from the cucumbers themselves – put the brisket on the fork – dip the brisket in a little bit of the olive oil – then dip the brisket in a little bit of the sauce around the mushrooms – then stab a mushroom – then, if I'm lucky, dip the mushroom and the brisket in a little bit of the barbecue sauce and put it in my mouth. I am not exaggerating – since I spent a good deal of time with my eyes down looking at my plate I have seen up to 13 moves with the fork before it goes in my mouth. Sometimes I just have to say – please just put it in my mouth. So while this example might be a bit humorous – and we certainly do try to have fun with the differences – it can be very tense for both my wife and for me. For me it is another one of those reminders that I have no control – even over what I eat. Because we do it so differently my wife often feels like she is not doing what I wanted her to do and is somehow or another inadequate. There is nothing further from the truth and you might not like the fact that I share this story. However, life with a person who has to be cared for is not easy. My wife would not have chosen to be a nurse – she knows very well her temperament and what she is good at by nature. To be put in this position and show the willingness, the love and the patience to take care of me is absolutely one of the greatest gifts of my life – and her biggest challenge.

Let me take a minute to talk about our friends and eating out with them. Every one of our friends knows how hard Karen works and how few meals she gets where she really just gets to talk, eat her meal by herself and not feed me. So these amazing people make sure when we go out that they take some of the burden off Karen. At first I found this difficult because it made my handicap so public. However, I soon realized that this was really a gift they were giving my wife and that it only made sense to go along with it and enjoy the ride. Now, all of our friends are more than willing to help but there are several that I really turn to when I am eating. I am only going to mention a couple of people who live here in Denver.

First is a friend who is the fastest eater west of the Mississippi. I am not kidding. In fact, it is not uncommon for his plate to be empty by the time my wife has prepared her plate and taken her first bite. So Pat is the perfect person to help me eat and as he is left-handed I try to sit on his right. Now here's the catch – his left hand shakes – sometimes it shakes a lot – and he is a talker – so I may not always be getting his full attention. So picture this – I have a nice bite of enchilada on the fork in Pats left hand – he is talking to someone over on the left side of the table not facing me – and I am bobbing and weaving trying to catch that fork with the enchilada on it and somehow get it in the middle of my mouth. I'm already tired. But I actually eat more and faster when I'm sitting next to this great and compassionate friend.

One other quick example – just a couple of weeks ago I was sitting at the table with my wife on my left and our friend Lana on my right. Lana made our dinner so much more enjoyable by helping me eat some of the food along with Karen so that she gets to take a few bites on her own. A very thoughtful and very kind gesture. Most importantly my wife had time off.

Again, these are only a couple of examples of our many friends who make sure my drink is in the right place, fill up a plate of food for me without being asked, take an appetizer off the plate and put it in my mouth and make sure that my needs are being met. I am a lucky man.

During the day it is nice to have something set out that I can snack on. My wife will put some almonds or cashews on a plate and put them on the counter for me. All I have to do is bend over and with my tongue pick up the item I want to eat. This is a very efficient process and very importantly to me gives me some independence. I don't have to have someone home and I can go in and get something to eat anytime. Sometimes there is candy there – sometimes there is cheese there – sometimes there are slices of an orange or an apple.

I have one other example of gaining some independence when I eat out. There are two restaurants/bars within 1 mile of my house so I'm able to walk to them by myself. I have gotten to know the bartenders and the wait staff and they are terrific. At one place they make boneless Buffalo wings and at the other place they make terrific chicken fingers. So here's the process. I have them put the Buffalo wings and/or the chicken fingers (they have to cut the chicken fingers up into smaller pieces for me) and place them on a piece of paper on the bar. I then have them put my drink with a straw next to the paper. I bend over just as I do when I eat my snacks at home and simply pick up the food with my tongue. They are just terrific and help me in every way including sometimes at the end of the meal when they have to wipe the extra buffalo sauce off the end of my nose. At the end of my meal I have them reach in my pocket and take out my wallet to pay them. I always try to tip more than is expected because I get such great service. Even though I do feel somewhat conspicuous eating this way in a public place – I have found that because I am on a first name basis with the bartenders the other patrons around me are usually very gracious and kind and I often have people offer to help. These are good days for me.

There are some tools to help you eat. During the transition of having full use of my hands and arms – to not having any use these limbs – there was a period of time where I was able to use knives, forks and spoons that are made specifically for people who lack function. Both the spoon and the fork have a very large handle and allow you to actually bend the head of the fork or the spoon in the direction that would make it easiest to put food in your mouth. I found these aides to be very helpful and I was able to use them for over a year. We have a store here in Denver called Youcan Toucan which has been a great resource for me in finding devices to make my life easier.

Here's a tip. When you're eating a doughnut or a bagel make sure to break it in half along the radius. If you eat it as a circle you're going to end up with either sugar or cream cheese on both of your cheeks. If you break it in half the way I suggested you'll have straighter pieces that are easy to put in your mouth and you won't end up with a mess.

Chapter 6

Technology, Friend or Foe

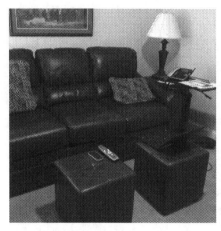 Here is a picture of what my command center looks like. Over a three-year period, with a lot of changes in my ability to function, we have come up with various strategies on how I can get things done during my day.

My command center is our den and includes four important technology features:

1. My laptop

2. My iPhone

3. My TV remote control

4. Our desk phone

I will explain a good bit and show pictures on how all this works for me. One of the really amazing things that I have found over the last three years is how few real electronic and/or mechanical devices exist for people who don't have the use of their arms and hands as a result of a neurological disorder. We have a world-renowned critical care facility here in Denver that won't even see me because my paralysis is not the result of an injury. At the University where I am a patient they have an Assistive Technology Department. What I learned is that there is no magic solution and technology. The therapist in this department has recommended a new mobile phone and potentially a new desk phone that can be voice-activated. It is important that we work collaboratively with our occupational therapist to identify those things that are most important to us and prioritize those things we want them to work on for us.

My Laptop – I was a business/telecommunications consultant at IBM for the past 15 years of my career. I love my work and I love my laptop. I like playing with spreadsheets – I like reading articles – I love researching things – and so when I knew I was going on disability and would no longer have the company laptop it was imperative that I get a light weight and easy to use laptop. I settled on a Lenovo because of the ties to IBM and my long time use of this technology.

The purpose of this book is to be practical – I have my laptop loaded with all the basic software I had before I retired. I like the Microsoft Suite of products and I know how to use – Word for documents and Excel for spreadsheets. I primarily use Explorer for the Internet, but I have both an MSN email that I share with my wife and Gmail for my personal

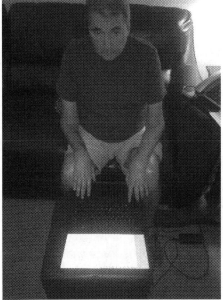

use. I can navigate between these very quickly. And perhaps the most important software for me is Dragon NaturallySpeaking. This speech to text software program has been very helpful. I am writing this book using Dragon. I do not expect perfection so I am not surprised that there are some challenges in using this – for example trying to fill in addresses on the address line or an email address can be very difficult for me. Also, most of the websites that I use that require usernames and passwords where all you see are dots instead of what you've

37

actually typed can be extremely difficult. (Complaint – websites should not make us change our passwords all the time – it makes it very difficult. Nuance, the company that owns the speech to text software should reconsider charging people to get a tutorial on how to use the software that they sell.)

Here is a picture of me sitting at my laptop – gravity is my friend. I position my hands on my knees – I raise my knees by lifting my heels off the floor – position my finger over the key I want to press – put my heel back down on the floor and that provides the necessary pressure on the key. I do the same thing to move the cursor – I move my knee to position my finger over the cursor – let it drop down – and move my finger by moving my knee back and forth in the direction I want the cursor to go – and then I lift it back up so that my hand is away from the cursor. I then lift my other knee and move my left index finger over the left cursor button and let my knee drop to depress it. (Wearing long pants sometimes works better than shorts as you can slide your hands more easily when there is not perspiration between your leg and your hand.)

When I'm doing simple things like reading the paper or Facebook or emails I am often able to just use the up and down arrows to navigate. This is the easiest for me to do – but when I have to do more complex things it isn't uncommon for me to have to stand up and sit down numerous times to position my finger over a key in order to depress it. If it is a long email address for example and I have to stand up to hit the shift key with my left finger and then drop my right middle finger over the appropriate character on the keyboard it can often take many attempts and over a period of time it is not uncommon for me to be sweating profusely having been worn out by the process. Here's the thing – I can do this – I can do this entirely by myself – I can communicate with my friends and family – I can research – I can communicate and I can feel pretty normal. There are so many who have advanced challenges who have to blow through tubes or blink their eyes in order to just accomplish a few characters on a page.

My iPhone – I don't know what I would do without Siri. I can press the button on the bottom of my iPhone using my technique of "stand up, bend over, depend on gravity" to provide the force necessary. If you know this technology you will know that you can simply speak and say "call mom and dad." With the iPhone that I have there is a bit of a challenge in pressing the speakerphone button after the call is dialed. I have to be very careful to position my thumb and/or my index finger over the speakerphone button and try to tap it. Sometimes I'm too late as this takes a long time and people will hang up. But all in all this is pretty good technology for me. Answering the phone can be more difficult. The reason is that you have to swipe the arrow at the bottom of the screen in order to get to the call when it rings. Swiping is not something I do very well. So I often miss calls. Again even if I'm successful at swiping and connecting to the call it still takes me some time to get to that speakerphone button and activate the speakerphone. It is not uncommon for people to hang

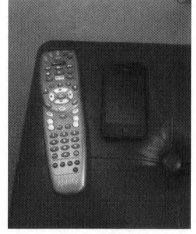

up on me prior to my completing all this. I wish that Apple would enable the phone to accept and dial calls completely hands-free. I've done lots of research and have still not found a desk phone or a mobile phone that is completely hands-free.

I love texting – simply by pressing the initial button I can say "text Allie" and I can keep talking and leave a text and then say "send" without ever having to touch anymore buttons.

You will see in the picture that I have my cell phone and my remote control for the television next to each other on a small ottoman. That seems to

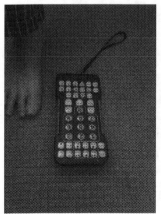

be a perfect height to be able to use both of these devices.

The remote control – this is also a very important part of my life. I watch a lot of news and I watch a lot of sports and I watch a good bit of the Discovery Channel along with my favorite CIS shows in the evening. For a long time I was able to hold the remote in my hand and position a finger or thumb over the key that I wanted to depress. I lost the ability to do anything with my fingers that relied totally on their own strength about eight months ago. Since I wrote my first draft of the book I have discovered two great new things at Comcast. We now have a remote control that is voice-activated which is a really nice feature. Only problem is you do have to hold down the button in order to activate it so that has its challenges. More brilliant is that Comcast has an assistive technologies group and all I had to do is place a call and they sent me this remote control that you see in the picture. It has all of the capability of the regular remote with very large buttons. Now all I have to do is set this next to my ottoman and I can perform all of these functions with my toes. This is truly an amazing capability for me and now I can channel surf again. I'm sure that this device would be very helpful for people with arthritis and site problems as well. Good for Comcast for providing this kind of device at no cost to their customers.

The desk phone – be sure not to just come over and use my desk phone. The reason is simple – I do everything with my tongue. It sits on the portable computer table next to where I sit. It has nice big keys and the speaker button that allows me to lean over and put my tongue on the speakerphone button to answer calls. When I'm making a call I carefully push in the numbers that I want to dial with my tongue as well. It's nice because it has a screen that shows whether or not I have input the proper numbers. After I input the numbers I simply tongue the speakerphone button and make my call. Karen sanitizes the phone every few days. I want this to be totally hands-free.

I'm sure there is a lot more I could say about all of this but one of the things that is important is that I have these most essential tools close by. I have them at a level that I can stand up or sit down and get my fingers positioned over the devices in order to activate them. By the way, the reason I can't operate the desk phone with my fingers is that it is too high up on the computer table for me to get my fingers above the phone. Remember, my arms don't move and I cannot lift them. So the height of my hands when I'm standing up is about mid-thigh.

There are a number of other things in my life that may be a little less technical but are no less important in order to be able to function with some degree of independence every day. Here are a couple of examples:

Light switches – we are fortunate to have a new home and have the types of light switches that we have installed. The switches allow me to just bump the switch with my forehead and turn the light in a room on or off. We have another wonderful device that we got at Costco that allows us to plug up to three lamps into a system that has a remote control. The remote control has three buttons – one for each light. I simply bend over and push the appropriate button with my tongue and I can turn on the table lamp. As you can imagine there's no way I can pull a string or turn a knob to do this so this was a great find by our friend Barb who "turned us on" to this great device.

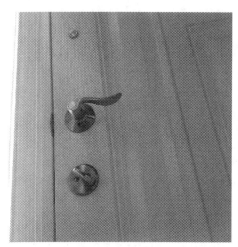

One final technology note for now and this is really important because it's mechanical not electronic and that is our door latches. This is not only a very important part of helping me meet my need for independence but it is also an incredibly important safety feature. I have to be able to get out of the house. I also need to be able to open the door to a room. Old-fashioned knobs just don't work. We have these wonderful door latches that allow me to swing my hand onto the top of the lever and by pressing my leg against my hand to press the lever enough to free it and then I make sure my hand is between the door and the lever and by pulling back with my whole body can open the door. It works! So if I have to get out of the house I can.

If I don't have the same kind of knob on both sides I'm not able to pull the door closed. Remember I can push but I generally cannot pull. I am able to pull the door open in the way I described in the previous paragraph if it is not too heavy and I sort of get my wrist between the door and the latch and then use my weight of my body to pull it open. But pulling the door shut in the same manner isn't as easy. So to get out of our house I go out the garage door using the method I just described – the door shuts itself behind me because it is on a self-closing hinge – push the garage door opener button with my tongue – then go outside and push the close button on the outside – wall-mounted keypad. Works like a charm! You won't be surprised to know that when I need to get back in the house I use my tongue to push in the numbers on the keypad, open the garage door and come in the way I left.

We have some wonderful HOA board members and when we moved in the community they accepted my request to change the knob system on the gates to our community with lever handles so that I would be able to come and go. Since then even these are difficult and I rely on the wonderful people, especially Tracy during the day, who maintain our security gate to let me in and out and always do so with a smile and a "how are you today Mr. Griffin, is there anything I can help you with?"

There were a lot of intermediate devices and tools that were helpful that I can no longer use. (My occupational therapist did a great job of keeping me informed about options.) We used spoons and forks and plates that were designed for people who had trouble eating and they were great for a time. So necessity is the mother of invention and that is never truer than for someone who has a part of their body that doesn't function. I'm sure many of you are much more creative/inventive than I am and have come up with many more techniques and aids to make your life more independent.

Chapter 7

Flexibility and Exercise

I cannot begin to tell you how important this is to me – to my sense of well-being and to my sense of independence. I've always loved exercising and since college cannot remember a time when I haven't done something. I wish my body looked more like I had done it all these years but without exercise I'm pretty sure I would be closer to 250 pounds than I am to the 180 to 190 pounds I weigh. This has also been an evolving journey for me as I started out losing strength and at first not knowing what was happening. Remember the bike wreck?

Let me take a moment to explain why this is so important to me. There are some very practical reasons for not having a big belly. When my belly gets too big I can't see the rings that I use to pull my pants zipper down. When it gets too big my wife has a harder time getting my pants buckled. When my stomach and my torso get too large it's much more difficult to pull a shirt over and position it. Those may not sound like a big deal to you but they are to me and they certainly are to my wife. So eating and drinking intelligently is important for me as well as exercise. I get up and I get down 100 times a day. Without a strong core I would never be able to turn over or to get out of bed or get up out of the chair since I no longer have my arms to help push me. It's incredibly important that you find a way to keep your core muscles strong and to try to keep your weight intact. (As I talk through this chapter I do so with the caveat that I know my doctor would want me to throw in. You cannot fatigue muscles that are affected by this disease. It just won't help – they cannot get stronger – they can only become more fatigued. My best example of this was when I was still able to use my arms to some extent and I was able to get a fork up to my mouth three maybe four times and on the fifth time I cannot lift it off the table. So be aware of your condition and what your body is telling you.)

Flexibility and range of motion are really important to maintain as much as you can. I've been given some great techniques and processes I can follow by my occupational therapist. But here is where I have an ace in the hole – my daughter Allie is both an educator and a licensed massage therapist. What a gift for me.

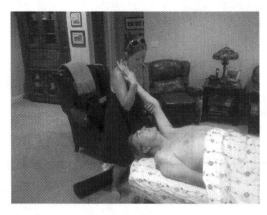

Every Saturday morning Allie comes over and sets up the massage table and gives me a great massage. More important than the massage is that she spends a good bit of time working on my range of motion. While lying on my back she extends my arm away from my shoulder and moves it as far back as she can. At the elbow she will move my forearm backwards and forwards applying pressure to the extent we see some progress. She does this with my wrists and my fingers as well. Allie is not only very capable but also very conscious of how much movement I can take and when I'm experiencing more pain than just discomfort and distinguishing between the two.

Since a person with drooping arms has a hard time maintaining good posture and that certainly is true of me my neck and shoulders can become very tense and also locked up. I lay on my back and Allie will move my head from the left side to the right side applying pressure, asking me to resist and then applying more pressure. This process does a lot to free up my neck muscles. The massaging of my neck and shoulder muscles is also extremely important to me and helps me, I believe, maintain good general health.

During the week my wife spends a lot of the time in the evening sitting next to me and doing flexibility exercises with my arms and hands as well. Just spreading out my fingers by placing her fingers between my fingers is one of the most comforting and useful flexibility exercises we do. I've mentioned previously, but when showering Karen will hold my hand up over her head by my wrist when she is both soaping me up, rinsing me off and finally drying me. This motion is so important on a daily basis and helps maintain both some flexibility and range of motion in my arms at the shoulder.

Both of these women are an amazing gift to me. Things that I just talked about are not easy to do physically and I think they take an emotional drain as well from the people who love you.

Physical Training – I love to go to the gym and I love to go for walks. They are two things that are not only good for me but also help me express my independence. (If you haven't caught on yet there's a theme here.)

Over the last three years Karen and I have walked hundreds of miles. We have adapted a vest that we put on when I walk and allows me to put my hands in the pockets of the vest and take the weight of my arms off my shoulders. (If you haven't thought of this please consider doing something to provide you a "sling like" relief for your arms.) Being out in the sunshine, walking and talking with my wife is not only great for my legs and my lungs but it is also great for our relationship and for my state of well-being.

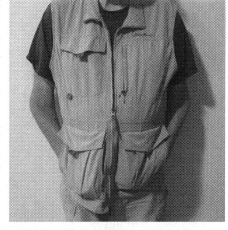

As I said before I love going to the gym and over the last couple of months I have been working with a wonderful physical trainer who has worked with me to utilize some of the equipment in the gym and to maintain as much fitness as is possible. So we concentrate on three things.

Aerobics – Core – Balance

Aerobics – this is actually pretty easy because when we arrive at the gym my wife puts me on the recumbent cycle – programs the machine for 45 to 60 minutes – puts it on "hills" – puts in my weight and sets it at level 10. I am able to spend almost an hour and work hard enough to work up a sweat and increase my heart rate. I get to do this while watching a couple of TVs that are set up over the cycles. (By the way, this is free. I have my supplemental health insurance through a company that has made the fitness gym available at no cost through their Silver Sneakers program.) Riding the recumbent cycle not only builds my lungs but also does a great job on my leg muscles and I believe that I am able to improve my posture while sitting on the seat.

Core – fitness trainers are constantly telling us how important our core is and if you lost the use of your arms or other parts of your body it seems that it is even more important and critical. If you think about what you do every day and you consciously take note of how you get in and out of the car, how you get out of bed how you stand up from the kitchen table and/or sit down – you will know that you use your hands and your arms constantly and you aren't even aware of it. So I have to make up with my core some of that leverage that I used to get with my arms. So there are a few simple things that my trainer has me doing that I can do by myself to improve my core.

1. I do three sets of 20 crunches on a slant board. This piece of equipment allows me to secure my feet underneath a foot bar and then lean back on the board and do crunches. This particular device has a very broad seat and I don't worry about falling off. I let my arms dangled to my side as I am unable to actually hold them in front of me and do the repetitions.

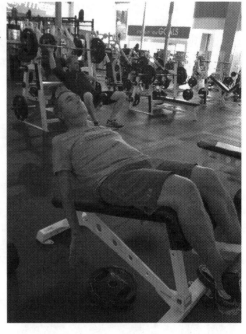

2. I do forward lunges. Not only does this work on my core but also works on my balance and my leg strength. Since I'm breathing hard when I'm finished I think it's also very good for my lungs. I simply find an open area like the gym itself and put 1 foot in front of the other and dip down and back up and repeat that forward motion about 25 times. It is a great exercise.

3. We've also worked out on various leg presses, both forward and back and other equipment in the gym. Unfortunately these pieces of equipment require someone to set the weights and so there needs to be someone around who is willing to help me. If there are people around I'll have them do this but they are not necessary for me to get a good workout.

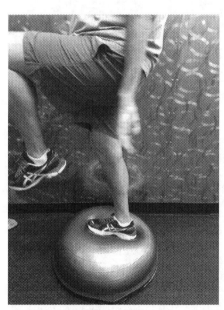

Balance – by now you know how much I rely on balance. There are a number of things that we do. First of all I want to point out that we put whatever piece of equipment we have next to a wall so that I have a place to bailout and catch myself. One of the simplest pieces of equipment is a step. This platform is about 12 inches off the ground and I just take turns moving from my right foot to my left foot stepping up on the platform. It's great for balance and it's also somewhat aerobic and strengthens my legs. The other device I use a lot is the bosu ball. This half sphere provides a real challenge for balancing. I do exactly the same thing I did with the platform but I make sure that I kick my opposite knee up as high as I can before I step off. I do 15 repetitions with my right leg and then 15 with my left leg. A great workout.

Those are all very simple and other than getting on the recumbent I don't really require any help and of course it is important to me to be as independent as possible.

One final exercise thought. I have a recumbent trike. Over the last 18 years I've been a very avid cyclist and taken lots of long rides both to enjoy my wife and my friends as well as to stay in shape. After the bike wreck I could not do that any longer so I bought a recumbent trike. That worked for a while but within about a year I was no longer able to safely pull on the hand brakes that allow you to stop. So I had a special trike built. The trike has coaster brakes so I simply have to pedal backwards and that will apply the brakes to my back wheels. I also had a special gearshift system put on the bike that really only has about six gears and that doesn't really matter anyway because I can't shift them on the move and so I leave it in one gear most of the time. The real trick now is holding on to the handlebars. On a recumbent trike the bars are next to my hips and of course I can't hold my arms up and I can't grasp the handle grips with my hands. So here's what we've come up with – we bought mountain bike gloves and had Velcro sewn into the palms of the gloves and also on the index fingers. The handlebars on recumbents have a small platform where my hands rest. 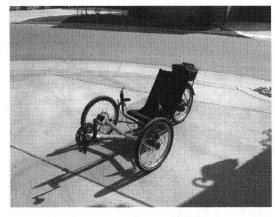 We put the other side of the Velcro on those hand rests and I "Velcro" my hands on to the handlebars. This works pretty well. I also cannot pull or push my arms anymore except a little bit by moving my shoulders. So now when I want to turn left I push my right knee against the right handlebar and that turns my tires to the left and do the opposite to turn to the right. My wife has become very concerned with my safety as I cannot really make a sharp left or right turn. In fact I have a bit of a hard time holding a straight line. So I think my time on my trike is limited but every couple weeks I go out to make sure I can still do it.

Conclusion

– Everyday Life – Lived Every Day

"There are three things that you should do every day – you should laugh – you should think – and your emotions should be moved to tears. If you do those three things you will have a heckuva day." Jimmy V-

My hope is that you experienced all three of these
things as you read this book.

"Today is Thursday, July 16, the 197th day of 2015. There are 168 days left in the year." Denver Post

I start every day by reading the paper – one of the features is keeping track of which day it is in the year and how many days are left. I've been using this now for three years to monitor my progress. Beginning in August 2012, I was acutely aware on a monthly basis of the loss of strength and function and by approximately that time in 2013 I had probably lost 70% – 75% of the strength in my arms and hands. During that same timeframe over the next 12 months I lost another 15%. During the past 12 months I have probably lost another 7 to 8%. So let me give you a glimpse of our lives on a given day. (I still have a couple of percent strength left in my hands/arms)

Earlier I described our morning and the number of tasks that my wife has to perform for me before 8 AM. In the previous chapters I talked about hygiene and going to the toilet and getting dressed and eating – obviously all of those things will take place today and took place yesterday and the day before that and will have to take place tomorrow and the next day.

49

Yesterday after we finished those tasks, and Karen washed my hair and got me dressed in my workout clothes – she buckled me into the front seat of the car and we drove over to my parents retirement home where we left our car, walked a mile and a half to a car dealership where my parents car was being serviced, picked up the car and drove it back to my parents, picked up our car and Karen buckled me back in, we drove to the 24 Hour Fitness location and Karen put me up on the recumbent trike and programmed it for me and she was able to go down and work with her personal trainer for an hour and not have to worry about me. Most of the time people are very gracious. But not always. I always think it's pretty obvious based on my posture and my droopy, skinny arms that there's something wrong with me but honestly a lot of people just don't notice. The other day at the club I was trying to use the leg press equipment. As a guy walked by who was about my age I asked him if he can give me a hand and he quickly said "no" – I said, "my arms and hands don't work could you please help me?" – "You're on your own buddy" and he walked away. That doesn't happen a lot but is a bit disheartening when it does.

When we arrived home we had a message from my mother that she needed a special cream from the pharmacy for my dad so we drove back over to the pharmacy and returned to their apartment to deliver the cream. Including having a quick lunch – showering and getting dressed before we went back over to my parents my wife has now performed another 25 to 30 tasks for me. Some as simple as buckling and unbuckling me in the car and others a bit more difficult like feeding me, showering me and getting me dressed. Remember it is barely past noon. (You know you are loved when your wife doesn't just care for you but also helps care for your elderly parents.)

When we get back home I come into the den and get my laptop up and running and find a message from Allie describing the work she's done on an ALS benefit that we are hosting on August 22. She is really amazing at not only trying to help physically but also do things that support us in awareness of the disease in trying to help people who are less fortunate than us. I also have read all my emails and I make reservations for a couple of nights in Vail with our best traveling buddies. I spent my afternoon watching golf and to make sure that the Denver Broncos get their wide receiver signed to a long-term contract.

About 4 o'clock I suggest maybe it's time for happy hour. So we get me in the car – head to a local watering hole – Karen comes around and opens my door and unbuckles me, – she closes the door behind me. People in the parking space next to us are staring intently at this process – I'm sure it looks odd to them. We go in and order a glass of wine and a couple of nibblies. I ask the waitress to please put a straw in my wine and she looks at me oddly and says "what, you can't drink fast enough without a straw?" It's late in the afternoon and sometimes you just get tired of trying to explain so we both just let it go and figure it will become self-evident sometime during the time we are there. As we are leaving the couple sitting next to us are leaving at about the same time and he graciously holds the door for both Karen and me, he nods and smiles. We actually get that a lot more than we get the negative looks. Please remember that when you see someone parking in a handicap spot who may not look challenged to you that they may have problems that you're not aware of and I encourage you to be gracious and give them the benefit of the doubt.

You get the picture – life becomes pretty routine for us. It isn't easy, and can be very difficult – in fact some days it just sucks. I think, for those who love and care for us it is difficult to watch and sometimes they don't know how to react. But all in all I believe that Karen and I would both say that we are thankful and blessed that we have the family we have supporting us – the friends and the neighbors that we have who support us – and that we have this life together.

There is a verse in the Bible that talks about being content in whatever state you find yourself. I have had a lifelong quest to achieve "peace" in my life. I've made a lot of progress on this lifelong quest. We've certainly been challenged more than we thought we would over the last three years but the idea that I can be content, even with life's difficulties, reminds me that I can have peace in my life.

Five Things I Would Love to be Able to Do Again

1. Put my arms around my wife and hold her
2. Get my penis out by myself at public restrooms
3. Feed myself
4. Pull my pants on and dress myself
5. Drive a car

Five of the Best Things People Have Said

"Mr. Griffin – I know you can't put your arms around me, but if I put your arms on my shoulders I can put my arms around you and give you a hug." Six-year-old student who I had the privilege of tutoring this year

"Grandpa – is there anything else I can do for you"
12-year-old grandson Garrett after helping program a phone for me

"I never hear you complain – your positive attitude has to have a major impact on how well you are doing!"
More than one of our friends

"Karen is amazing – you really are the luckiest man in the world."
All of our friends and all of my children

"If you think losing your hands is going to cause me to go easy on you on the golf course you have another thing coming"
Ridley and Pat

One final quote "grandpa – you can't move your hands but I can move mine" three-year-old Ivy

Special Acknowledgments

Always to Allie who checks in everyday and shows her love and concern not only with her actions and generosity but also with her tears.

To our son-in-law Jeff who took most of the pictures and is such a great human being. To sons Rex, Slade and his wonderful family who go out of their way to come this way and help us keep our homes repaired. Rex lives in Hong Kong and Slade in Tennessee – when I say they go out of their way – they really go out of their way.

To Kristi and her family– we could have never gotten her mother out of the old house without Kristi's ability to get her mom moving and everyone pitching in to make it happen. Son Tyson – who never fails to express his love. Reid at Sunbrook golf course in St. George always greets us with a smile and an "I can get you off the first tee in about 10 minutes." Our friends and neighbors – who have always given us hope – encouragement and support – Lana and Ridley and Pat and Linda have been there from the start. Friends Barbara and Sandy who always seem to know when it's time to give Karen a call and just go to lunch with the girls. The irrepressible Triona who last night fed me my chips and guacamole. And of course my best friend Gary who every couple weeks drives all the way down from Boulder just to spend the day with me so Karen can take off and play golf with the girls. I cannot express how much I appreciate these acts of kindness. I cannot express how much I love these friends. Kari and all the wonderful first-graders she teaches at Arrowhead Elementary who let me work with them and try to help them read. Our wonderful Aussie friends Tom and Judy who are so generous in every way to us. And to our great friends from Pennant Hills Golf Club in Sydney Australia who have raised over $2 million in support of the people with MND. And to all of those – all of you – who contributed to the ice bucket challenge.

<u>All of you are the blessings we experience every day in our lives!</u>

Finally – to my Mom and Dad – I just wish that when I asked my dad "can you get my penis out so that I can pee?" He would rethink his response of –

"I can't find it!"

About the Author

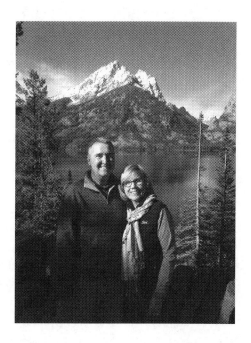

I was diagnosed approximately three years ago with a motor neuron disease that has left me without the use of hands and arms. This progressive disease started simply with the loss of the ability to clip my fingernails and has progressed to the point where I'm completely dependent on my wife for my daily needs. As I went through the process of losing functions, it became more and more apparent to me that I needed to develop some techniques, processes, tools, and capabilities that would allow me as much independence as possible and make it as easy on my caregiver as possible daily. This with this in mind that I decided to write a book about what life is like both physically and emotionally for family.

In the book I try to describe what a day in the life of a person whose hands don't work actually looks like. As a shared the manuscript with a number of friends who spend a good bit of time with us—I constantly got the comment—"I had no idea how many challenges the two of you face every day." "We knew it was difficult but you often handle did so well that we didn't see all the things that you do as a couple in the background." There's really nothing more personal than all the things that we do on a daily basis that enable us to get up and go out and be in public. What I hope I am able to do in this book is to provide people some how-to ideas on how to adapt to losing the use of hands and arms. Certainly in addition I want you to feel some of the feelings that we do.

I spent most of my career in the telecommunications and IT consulting industries. My career was most fulfilling, having served for over eleven years as an executive with one of the regional Bell operating companies and then getting an opportunity to finish my career as an international consultant with the IBM Corporation. In addition to that, I had the honor to teach both the secondary and college levels and serve as a vice-chancellor in what was then the Oregon State system of higher education.

My wife, Karen, and I have been married for the last eighteen years and have been able to combine our families that now include five children along with their spouses and a combined thirteen grandchildren. We've lived most of our married life in Denver, Colorado, but had the wonderful opportunity to spend two-plus years in Sydney, Australia, where we developed lifelong friends who we have added and infiltrated with her fabulous friends here in Colorado. We've been fortunate the last three years to have a second home in St. George, Utah, where it is warm in the winter and I don't have to worry about slipping on the snow and ice.

Printed in the United States
By Bookmasters